M000211389

BODY
FIXX

BODY
FIXX

A Positive Guide for Losing
Weight with Confidence

DR. HOPE WATTS, MD, FAAFP

publish
your gift

BODY FIXX

Copyright © 2021 Hope Watts

All rights reserved.

Published by Publish Your Gift®

An imprint of Purposely Created Publishing Group, LLC

No part of this book may be reproduced, distributed or transmitted in any form by any means, graphic, electronic, or mechanical, including photocopy, recording, taping, or by any information storage or retrieval system, without permission in writing from the publisher, except in the case of reprints in the context of reviews, quotes, or references.

Unless otherwise indicated, scripture quotations are taken from the Holy Bible, King James Version. All rights reserved.

Printed in the United States of America

ISBN: 978-1-64484-384-0 (print)
ISBN: 978-1-64484-383-3 (ebook)

Special discounts are available on bulk quantity purchases by book clubs, associations and special interest groups. For details email: sales@publishyourgift.com or call (888) 949-6228. For information log on to www.PublishYourGift.com

To my brother Courtney, my sister Elaine, and my cousin Pam, who have prayed for me, supported me, and encouraged me in my endeavors.

To my mother, who has passed but would have definitely encouraged me to write my book.

To my dear friend Antinetta Vanderhorst, who has walked with me through various life journeys. Who has prayed and given encouragement and advice.

To Helen Hopkins, who is a fellow author, who has encouraged me to write a book for several years. Who has prayed and given encouragement and advice.

TABLE OF CONTENTS

INTRODUCTION

Are you tired of trying to lose weight? Have you tried every new diet that has come out? Many diets promise weight loss but you find that you have not achieved any weight loss.

Sonia was very active in sports as she was growing up. She was actually a track star as a teenager, and she continued this on through college. After having her last child (third) she just could not lose that "baby fat." She tried many of the popular fad diets. Many gave fabulous, raving reviews. She even Googled a few to see if they were worthwhile. There were many comments about how effective they were. The last diet she tried lasted for three weeks. It helped with her constipation, but true weight loss was not achieved. In her mind, she relegated this to another failed attempt at weight loss. What makes matters worse, she overheard her kids saying, "She's always on a diet." When her husband asked her about going to her high school reunion, she gave him a very vague answer. In her heart of hearts, she had already decided that she would probably not go to the school reunion due to her weight. This is due to the fact that her last diet did not work out as she had planned. Deep within she wondered if she would ever lose weight!

Yes, weight loss can be achieved. With the right approach, including food choices and fitness, you can achieve your weight loss goals. Diets give a sense of finite use. In actuality, some can spur lifestyle changes that benefit you and your family lifelong. Exercise done on a regular basis will give you extra energy and allow you to sleep better. Weight loss will help decrease your risk factors for many chronic diseases. You will also have a sense of well-being knowing that you've done this for your health and to be around for your family and watch your children as they grow up.

In my book you will learn that there are many barriers to weight loss. These will need to be addressed so that you will prevent another unsuccessful attempt. Mindset is a new concept, but it can make the difference in how well you do. Negative mindsets prevent you from reaching your goals. We do have diets in the book. Some of them, like the Mediterranean diet, can be used long-term to bring about permanent lifestyle changes. Exercise—both cardio and strength training—is reviewed to give you a framework as to how much you need to do. We also go into the benefits of exercises. We even delve into how to maintain your lifestyle habits even when going out to the restaurant. Additionally, there is information on food additives and preservatives. These are but a few of the items we will discuss.

My Story

I have always wanted to work in healthcare, but I realized that I truly wanted to become a medical doctor after I got into undergraduate school. I went to the Medical College of Pennsylvania in Philadelphia for my medical education, and I did my residency at St. Francis Hospital in Wilmington, Delaware, in family practice. Throughout my medical education I found that I was able to burn up all the calories I was consuming.

After working a few years in Delaware, I moved to Charlotte, NC, to work at an established practice. Within a few years, I was informed by my manager that I was nominated for the physician of the year award. I also became NCQA-certified in diabetes. This was sponsored by the National Committee for Quality Assurance. After passing the requirements, you are put on their national website of experts in diabetes. The pharmaceutical company Novartis gave me an award for selling the most Diovan (hypertension drug) in Charlotte at the time. During the earlier years of my career, I managed to eat healthy and exercise to keep my weight down.

As my career progressed, I was seeing more patients and had more responsibilities. Family practice is what I enjoyed; I loved seeing the variety in patients. Eventually we started using an electronic medical record in our office. I saw my ability to control my environment decrease and noticed that my whole life was geared around the electronic medical record. I found that I was sitting for long hours. Eating on the go a lot more. On most days, I did not get enough sleep. With long hours at work and decreased sleep, this made it difficult for me to get up and get my exercising in.

Gradually my weight was creeping up. Yes, I was very stressed! At this point I decided to ask my doctor for help. I was told that with a very stressful career and erratic hours I simply would not be able to lose weight.

I knew that I should be able to lose the weight. Realizing that I needed a different approach, I adjusted my schedule at work. I started preplanning my meals and snacks that I took to work. I worked hard to get adequate sleep nightly. Getting on my exercise bike most days of the week was a must. I started to lose weight after a few months. This showed me that working on weight loss when weight gain is first noticed can give you a head start on decreasing your weight. I have been able to maintain my weight within a few pounds despite my hectic, stressful career.

PART 1

What Is the Right Approach to Weight Loss?

CHAPTER 1

IS THIS YOUR SEASON?

You have always wanted to lose weight for as long as you can remember. You've had many false starts and you've done a lot of yo-yo dieting galore. Often you find it difficult to get in your exercise due to taking care of your husband and children, work responsibilities, and taking care of elderly parents. Or there just never seems to be enough time.

Last month you were finally able to be at your family reunion. You were really excited to see everyone. Of course, Aunt Sadie was there giving out her opinions. She did not mince any words when you came by. "Have you gained more weight? I almost didn't recognize you." Did she really have to say that in front of everyone? Your husband did not have much else to say. Actually, you think he seemed to be grinning.

You have enjoyed participating in the weight challenges at work; there's always a lot of excitement associated with these challenges. In fact, you won last year. You received $150! The goal was to lose 10 pounds and you exceeded that goal. Your clothes were fitting better and you had more energy. But in a matter of months, the weight came back and a sense of dissatisfaction crept in. "Why can't I be persistent in reaching my weight loss goal?" You often ask yourself. In your mind you cannot figure out why this keeps happening. You have many friends that have gone on to slimmer selves and are enjoying it. And of course, they're very happy about their accomplishment.

Cassandra, your neighbor down the street, worked out with you last year. Cassandra went walking with you almost every day in the summertime. She had weight loss goals and you were able to exercise most of the time with her. But September came and the kids had to go back to school, and you realized that there were many things you had to do while they were in school. This made it hard to keep the exercise going with Cassandra. This was yet another time that you could not continue with your weight loss.

Dieting or changing your lifestyle soon became something to avoid. You felt like you were not able to accomplish anything. In the past you had always started strong but somewhere in the middle of your journey you got sidetracked or distracted. As it turns out, you have never really stuck with any weight loss program or lifestyle change program to reach your desired goals. Losing weight had become a term to avoid at all costs. You would tell yourself "This is not for me." You no longer wanted to try. "Some people are just born big," you would say. You had resolved yourself to the notion, "Why do I need to lose weight anyway?"

Does this sound like you? Some people believe in the school of thought that what you don't know can't hurt you. This is the furthest thing from the truth. There may be many conditions that may not be apparent at first but will be diagnosed at a later date. Many of these conditions are associated with excess weight. Wouldn't you want to be proactive and do your part? If you knew you could improve your life, wouldn't you want to take advantage of the tools available to you?

Let's look at some of the issues we need to consider when we are undertaking weight loss or lifestyle goals.

Undertaking weight loss and lifestyle goals can be very beneficial. But it takes persistence to stick with the goals, especially when you don't see any movement. Motivation for completing this type of task comes from deep within. It could be that you saw something on TV. There are many infomercials that draw people in to pay a lot of money, but they give no lasting result. Sometimes motivation is spurred by another person's unfortunate death. This can happen as a result of the untimely death of a coworker or family member. There are other people who are motivated because some major event happens in their life or someone else's life. It could be that these people were overweight and word got to you that the reason for their misfortunes was related to their weight. Additionally, you may decide on your own that you want to be healthier and be able to be around your children and your grandchildren and have time to enjoy them. Making up your mind that you're going to change your lifestyle, which includes weight loss and other changes, is half the battle.

Weight loss may include changing a lot of old eating habits that are not productive. This may include switching to healthier foods. This may also mean that you will need to decrease and finally stop your visits at the fast-food restaurants. Or grabbing snacks from the snack machine. It may also mean getting rid of those extra sugary beverages. And this of course may mean you'll have to replace it with water or some other beverage that is not harmful. Additionally, you may have to start exercising on a regular basis. This may mean putting time aside to get in 30 to 45 minutes most days of the week (1). I used to recommend to persons that are endeavoring on their weight loss or lifestyle goals that they need to take one step at a time and gradually build a schedule that includes some of these recommendations. This is so people do not feel frustrated in trying to do too many different things at one time. The ultimate goal is that you can chart success no matter what part of your weight loss/lifestyle change you are endeavoring to do.

Distractions come in many forms and can prevent us from being successful in many endeavors including weight loss. The more major the life event, e.g., financial issues and marital issues, the more it can impact your ability to concentrate on your weight loss goals. Talk with your doctor about some of these issues because together you may decide that doing smaller changes may be appropriate. These steps may include incorporating the correct amount of water or getting in your 10,000 steps in per day, whereas larger changes such as being on a specific eating plan and setting specific days for exercise may be harder to accomplish.

Often, reaching lifestyle goals takes a lot of fine-tuning along the way. You may want to lose several pounds all at once. But that may not be realistic in the long term. You may be overestimating what you can do. To change this, it may mean that you will have smaller goals for shorter periods of time so that you can eventually reach those long-term goals. Eventually you will reach your long-term goals, but you'll need to be a little bit more patient. It may also mean that you need to change the type of exercise you're doing. It may also mean you'll need to change the days that you exercise and the type of exercise equipment. This requires that you allow yourself time to get adjusted to these new changes. Sometimes it's also helpful if you have a large amount of patience. Remember that for long-term success, it is worth taking the time to build a good foundation.

Sometimes emotional problems can create situations where you are not mindful about your eating. In this case, I would have to say that it is more likely that the emotions are controlling you. If you have anxiety or depression or some other mental health concern it may be hard to stay focused. Additionally, you may find yourself doing a lot of emotional eating. The majority of the time when this happens, it means that you're eating a lot of carbohydrates. Generally, they are in the category of empty calories. Empty calories include cakes, cookies, candy, chips, pastas, and breads to name a few. This may halt progression of your weight loss endeavors. Talk with your doctor about what you're experiencing emotionally. This may mean that you will need to see a counselor face-to-face or online, depending on how your insurance provides for it. Taking the time to explore how you're feeling is probably not high on your list if you want to lose weight. But it has been shown time and time again that one has to be focused and persistent in order to have lasting results. Doing this at the very beginning of your weight loss endeavors will enhance the success that you will achieve.

With any major endeavor, you do need a support system. You will need this support to get you through the difficult times. They will encourage you to be your best self and take hold of the vision that you have for yourself. This support may be in the form of an accountability partner or a weight loss group. Accountability partners will call when it is time to exercise (they may even exercise with you). You may also consider an online weight loss group or consider a certified health coach.

If you have given thought and are willing to work step-by-step on the topics we have just discussed, you may be on your way to starting a successful weight loss program. I like to call them lifestyle changes. If you have the attitude that you're going to lose a lot of weight and then go back on the same diet you were eating before, you will not be able to keep the weight off. If you approach your lifestyle change as lifelong, you will have permanent lasting weight loss success. Remember, "Rome wasn't built in a day." Your lifestyle changes will take time for you to adjust to them. Remember to give yourself time to reevaluate challenges so that you can make accurate corrections. Some lifestyle changes are easier than others. Remember to be kind to yourself. It takes constant practice to create a new habit. Keep a diary so you can reward your good behaviors. Of course corrections are going to be inevitable, but they will bring you closer to your goals.

CHAPTER 2

WHAT IS MINDSET?

There are many situations in life where we do not feel like we are moving forward. Weight loss can seem like this. We've tried many different types and versions of diets, but we do not seem to be getting to our goal weight.

Let me ask you a few questions:

1. Have you tried multiple diets and found that nothing has worked?

2. Is there some failure in your past that keeps you from moving forward with your weight goals?

3. Do you start strong on your weight loss quest, and as life stressors come about, do you abandon your goal yet again? Has this been happening all too often?

4. Does this sound like you? You joined the weight loss challenge at your workplace. You really worked hard at getting to the weight they had challenged you to reach. You won the $200 that they offered if you lost the 25 pounds. You felt triumphant at this time! But within a few months, however, you gained all the weight back again.

5. Does this sound like you? You decided to buy a treadmill. It has all the bells and whistles like you saw on TV. It is pricey but you wanted to look like the people on TV. Before long, the treadmill became a place for you to hang your clothes. It is not a place for exercise as you envisioned.

If this sounds like you, you may have a challenge with your mindset or how you think about weight loss.

Let us digress and give you a fuller picture of what mindset means.

Mindset

Mindsets are our beliefs about our basic qualities, i.e., intelligence, personality, or talent. Mindsets are also attitudes that manage our actions and interactions with the world. They are a way of thinking about the world and what we believe we can accomplish or cannot accomplish.

If we do not have a positive mindset, we hinder many of the goals we have set out for ourselves including weight loss.

Negative Thoughts

Let's discuss negative thoughts. Negative thoughts can be a part of our mindset. We can hold these thoughts in our minds and not really know what kind of damage they are doing.

Statistics show that the average person has about 12,000 to 60,000 thoughts per day. Of these thoughts:

- 80% are negative
- 90.5% are repetitive thoughts (2)

As you can see, negative thoughts or a negative mindset can be a major hurdle to overcome for many people who want to lose weight. Many start with lofty goals only to see themselves sabotage their journey with negative mindset or thought patterns. Most of the time they are not aware of these habits.

Overcoming deep-rooted negative thoughts or mindsets as we have stated can really hold you back, but once you have identified what they are and understood the importance of a positive mindset, you can change everything in your perspective and the goals you have for your weight loss.

The single best way to improve your health is to improve your mindset and your perspective. It will change what you believe you can accomplish. The way we think determines what we do, the excuses we tell ourselves, and the choices we make.

Some recent research about mindset shows that the more dissatisfied women feel about themselves and their bodies, the less likely they will participate in exercise. Additionally, psychologists stress that how you see yourself and your core mindset or attitude predicts your action or your inaction.

So, your attitude determines your altitude (how much you are going to succeed). The Bible verse that comes to mind about the situation is Proverbs 23:7, "For as he thinketh in his heart, so is he."

The good news is that many people can achieve their weight loss goals by changing their attitudes or their mindset. Fortunately, our minds are so flexible that we can train ourselves to do various new tasks.

Here are some suggestions for developing a different way of approaching weight loss and in doing so, changing your mindset:

Change Goals to Attainable Goals

We will need to change some of the goals we set for ourselves. Some things we can control ourselves and that makes it easier for us to have some success. Some of these goals are easier to accomplish, such as decreasing the number of sugary drinks you have on a daily basis. Eating less of those snack foods you know are not good for you. This may include chips, candy, and cookies. Taking these small steps may make it easier to get in five servings of fruits and vegetables a day. Other goals will get easier as you have small successes. Try getting in eight hours of sleep a day; also get eight to ten glasses of water in per day (3).

Gravitate to Positivity

1. Surrounding yourself with positive people
   Being around positive people promotes encouragement for your emotional health and a healthy environment.

This may give you the needed support to start out on your weight loss journey.

2. Surrounding yourself with others who have a common weight loss goal

These people tend to push you forward beyond your limits. They will remind you of the goals that you have set. They will help you meet or exceed the goals you have set out.

Your support system will help you focus on goals you can do every day such as achieving 10,000 or 15,000 steps a day. The people that support you will encourage you to not place restrictions on the time it takes to lose your goal of 40 pounds. (This can create extra pressure and extra stress and it may be setting you up for failure.)

Give yourself kudos for achieving your daily goals—all this encouragement will pay off in the end.

Recurring Negative Thoughts

You may find that there are some negative thoughts that don't seem to go away. Some of these thoughts could be from childhood or from a failure you may have experienced. Maybe you have identified these thoughts but you still aren't able to get rid of them.

1. Some people are able to decrease these thoughts or stop them altogether by doing positive affirmations every day.

2. Some people distract themselves by playing music or getting involved in other activities that prevent them from thinking about themselves (this is where having positive people helps you move through this).

3. Still, others find these thoughts to be recalcitrant and they are not able to deal with them (3). Some may need a health and wellness coach to walk them through some other solutions that may help them.

When Should I Step on My Scale?

The answer: Very infrequently

Many people find that they want to know how much they have lost. They check the scale frequently only to find out they have not lost many pounds at all. This can be a very discouraging activity for lots of people (3).

People can often tell if they have lost weight, especially from how their clothes are fitting. Also, many people can notice how much weight you have lost just by looking at your body proportions.

It is good to have a scale at home, but only check it once a week or every two weeks.

True Beauty Is What We Carry Inside

Do you spend a lot of your time looking to social media, your favorite singer, or Hollywood stars for your identity? Many of them have the money to spend to make sure certain wrinkles are gone or certain flabbiness has been taken care of. Do not spend your time comparing yourself to them.

Be kind to yourself— think of all the beauty you have inside. Think of your generosity to others in need. Think of how you help people who are less fortunate than yourself. This is where true beauty is.

Do not compare yourself with others. You are unique and there is no one else like you.

CHAPTER 3

DO I WANT LIFESTYLE CHANGES OR DIETS?

There are many diets that you can look into as you go on your weight loss journey. Let's face it, many people begin multiple diets but do not accomplish anything. Some diets are just too restrictive to continue lifelong. Others may not be the right fit for your lifestyle and for you or your family. However, you can choose the one that works best for you. With the aid of a health coach, you may be even more successful than before. Finding what fits may help you make permanent lifestyle changes. Let's look at some of the most popular diets and see what you can expect.

The Mediterranean Diet

This diet is inspired by the eating preferences of those living near the Mediterranean Sea. It is one of the most popular diets in the U.S., Canada, and Australia. This diet stresses eating plenty of fresh fruits, veggies, and white meat (fish, chicken, and turkey). Also, it stresses the use of olive oil, nuts, whole grains, and legumes. It is very well-known for its herbs and spices. You are allowed to drink red wine with dinner (this is included in the diet suggestions).

Things to think about: eating a lot of fresh veggies, cheese, chicken, and fish is very healthy and nutritious. It can be expensive to maintain in some parts of the country. I still believe that there are creative ways to get around some of these hurdles. Additionally, if you want to lose weight on this diet, you are still going to need to exercise and decrease the number of calories. Another thing to consider is the fact that there are no processed foods involved here and there are no fast foods involved in this diet. So, most of the food would need to be cooked. You would need to have training if you didn't know how to cook some of these foods. This is by far one of the healthiest diets and pretty simple to start (4).

The Paleo Diet

This has become a very popular diet recently. This diet claims that modern foods have evolved much faster than our bodies. This causes a state of chronic illness. The diet recommends eating the way that Paleolithic humans may have eaten. It consists of grass-fed beef, seafood, fresh fruits, and vegetables. It does allow eggs, nuts, seeds, and healthy oils. These healthy oils include walnut, avocado, coconut, and olive oils. It also avoids some very common foods, thus making for a very restrictive diet. We find that foods such as sugar and refined vegetable oils are not in the diet. You will find that processed foods, which include juices, sodas, and fast foods, are not included. This diet also avoids processed cereals, whole grains, and legumes including peanuts. Dairy is also not allowed.

Good points about the paleo diet: it is definitely a very healthy diet. There are no processed foods, but it is high in protein. You will definitely feel full for a longer period of time. And this will avoid those cravings that we often have when we're on those highly processed foods. The nutrients from plants, vegetables, and healthy oils are anti-inflammatory. This diet may help with inflammatory diseases.

Things to think about with this diet: the diet lacks vitamin D and calcium. Vitamin D and calcium supplements would have to be taken on a daily basis. Also, vegetarians would have a hard time with this diet. This diet does not allow beans or dairy. This diet is very restricted for most people and many will not be able to stay on the diet for long periods of time. Also, this diet can be pricey because most of the foods are specialty foods and you would have to go to special stores to buy these foods (4).

The Ketogenic Diet

This diet emphasizes weight loss through using healthy fats instead of carbohydrates. The goal is to quickly move into healthy fats so that ultimately you will feel fuller with fewer cravings. This diet will boost your mood and mental focus and increase your energy. By decreasing the carbs that you eat and increasing the good healthy fats (coconut oil, avocado oil, and olive oil) you will get to a state of ketosis. The body then breaks down dietary and stored fats to produce ketones. Your body then relies on fat instead of sugar for energy. This diet is different than other low-carb diets because it has extreme carb restrictions. Some diets allow only 20 net carbs or less per day. The deliberate shift into ketosis is what sets this popular diet apart from other low-carb diets such as the Atkins diet (5).

A recent study in the Journal of the American Medical Association came to these conclusions. They found that many people felt less hungry on this high-fat (good fat) diet, so many naturally reduced their overall caloric intake. Diabetic management showed improvement (5). Insulin sensitivity went down and the blood sugar control for people following the ketogenic diet was much improved.

Good points: this diet helps people have good weight loss, but many people will need to educate themselves about the amount of carbs and fat that is recommended for this diet. Exercise should be included in this diet also to increase the amount of weight loss. It is suggested that people exercise a minimum of 30 minutes a day. It is also advisable to get one of the carb apps. Also, get a book on the ketogenic diet so that you can follow its recommendations.

Things to consider: it can be expensive purchasing grass-fed beef, butter, and pasteurized chicken. You may have to order from a nearby farm to get cheaper prices. If you buy local, you are assured that it is fresh and without a lot of pre-servatives. Buying in bulk may save you money. You would probably need to expand your list of recipes to be consistent with the keto diet. Additionally, you may have to purchase the olive oil and avocado oil in bulk. Many food stores do offer home delivery for these items.

Weight Watchers (WW)

This diet has always been very popular. Weight Watchers has had numerous Hollywood stars that have lost weight with their programs. It is also a very flexible diet and there are no foods off limits; it just really depends on the plan that you choose. Weight Watchers has now rebranded themselves as WW. The new program has three plans. Most of the plans are just older plans that they have revised. The program has smart points and these points are designed to get your eating healthier. Here is an example: as calories and saturated fat increase, so do the smart points. If you want a leaner diet, then your smart points are lower. You must stay within the daily target of points. You can spend the smart points on food or beverages. You can track these points on the WW app. This app will allow you to track your smart points budget and how much exercise you do, and you can add on personal coaching if you so desire.

Even though Weight Watchers is known for diets, this new revised WW is more like a lifestyle maintenance program. The plans have recipes custom-made for you. The new emphasis is on incorporating regular exercise based on national recommendations and new mindset strategies that have proven to bring about behavioral changes (6).

Good points: The program is very flexible and it's easy to change your habits. You don't have to purchase prepackaged foods. Exercise will get you fitness points. And you will get points for engaging a mindfulness teaching.

Things to consider: all types of plans have a starting fee (depending on the plan). All the plans have access to digital content. Additionally, you can elect to have one-on-one support from a coach. Everyone has access through the WW app. Expect to learn how to shop and cook for healthy foods.

Clean Diet

Suppose you could lose weight without counting calories. Suppose you didn't have to have a whole lot of restrictions as you make your lifestyle choices. Then the clean diet may be for you. This diet allows you to eat lean protein, whole grains, good fats, and fresh fruits and vegetables. You're even allowed to eat small meals about six times a day. If you are consistent with the diet, it will increase your metabolic rate and it is estimated that you may lose about three pounds a week (this is an estimate of course because everyone is different). You may also have a lot of energy and may not be as hungry. The clean diet does not ban food groups but it recommends controlled portions (7).

They have specific guidelines on what you should be eating to maximize and optimize this diet plan. They recommend that you should eat breakfast within one hour of getting up. Also they recommend eating lean protein with complex carbohydrates with every meal including snacks. Healthy fats should be eaten two to three times a day. The water recommendation is two to three liters a day and at least four to five servings of fruits and vegetables a day.

As you would expect with diets that stress high nutrition, processed foods are eliminated. This includes white flour, white sugar, sodas, and juice. Foods with preservatives and added chemicals are also eliminated. Fat such as trans fat and saturated fats are not recommended. Exercise is also a cornerstone of this diet. The recommendation is to do cardio at least five to six times a week. The timeframe spent in this exercising ranges from 30 minutes to 45 minutes (6).

Things to consider: since most of the foods do not have preservatives, you may find that the food is not staying fresh very long. You may need to shop more frequently. There is also a lot of time commitment for exercising as recommended by the plan. You have to consider how much time you can put into exercising. Overall this plan does have high nutritional value and flexibility and can be used as a lifestyle change indefinitely.

CHAPTER 4

HAS ANYONE THOUGHT ABOUT FASTING?

We are now going to turn our attention to a newer type of lifestyle approach called intermittent fasting. We're also going to look at the pros and cons of this type of lifestyle. Fasting is not new. Many religions practice this. These groups include Christianity, Judaism, Buddhism and Islam. In its traditional forms, it usually means fasting for at least one day without eating. More often, however, people will fast one meal a week or from sunup to sundown.

We will now discuss some of the basic types of fasting that help with weight loss. There are many studies in humans that show that it is safe and incredibly effective for weight loss. As with all diets, you need to have a concrete plan and stick with it.

The definition of intermittent fasting is an eating pattern that cycles between periods of fasting and eating. It is currently very popular in the health and fitness communities.

There are several types of intermittent fasting, or IF. The first type is called the 16/8 method. With this type of intermittent fasting you are restricting your calories daily, between eating for 8 hours and then fasting for the rest of the day (which is 16 hours).

The second type of intermittent fasting is called "eat, stop, eat." It involves fasting for 24 hours once or twice a week. So, to complete this plan you would skip dinner on the day you decide to start the fast, and then resume your eating on the next day at dinner time.

The third type of intermittent fasting is called the 5:2 diet. In essence, you consume only 500 to 600 calories on two non-consecutive days of the week, but you eat normally on the other five days.

By reducing your caloric intake in any of these methods you should lose weight. The downside is that some people overcompensate and eat more food during their eating periods. The last two methods are harder for people to do on a regular basis. The 16/8 method appears to be the one used the most. It is easier to sustain and this can be a 7:00 AM to 3:00 PM time frame or a 1:00 PM to 9:00 PM time frame depending on the person's schedule (8).

What Do I Eat on This Diet?

During the times when you're not eating, you can drink water and zero-calorie beverages such as black coffee and tea. During the eating periods, you should strive to eat a healthy, balanced, nutritious diet. The most highly recommended diet is the Mediterranean diet. Eating high-calorie foods from your favorite fast-food restaurant is not going to help with weight loss. Additionally, processed foods and snacks are not recommended (8).

There is definitely an adjustment period for this type of lifestyle. Research shows that it can take two to four weeks before the body becomes accustomed to intermittent fasting (1). Sometimes you may feel hungry or cranky while getting used to the new routine. People who make it through this period tend to stick with it because they notice they are feeling better (8).

What Are the Intermittent Fasting Health Benefits?

Of course, the number one benefit is weight loss. Intermittent fasting can help you lose weight in the belly or the muffin top without conscientiously restricting calories.

If you are practicing intermittent fasting, you can lower your blood sugar about 3 to 6%. Intermittent fasting also lowers insulin levels by 20 to 30%, which would protect you from type 2 diabetes. This information is very helpful if your doctor has told you that you're moving into prediabetes (8).

If your family has a history of heart attack and stroke, intermittent fasting may reduce the bad LDL cholesterol. This is one of the risk factors for heart disease. Blood pressure and the resting heart rate are also improved.

For persons with a history of Alzheimer's disease in their family, intermittent fasting can boost verbal memory in adults. It is theorized that this form of lifestyle change may be protective against Alzheimer's disease. If you are using the Mediterranean diet, eating whole foods and avoiding preservatives and extra sugar may be part of this protective nature with intermittent fasting (8).

For many who are into physical performance, maintaining muscle mass is very important. It has been shown that men who have fasted for 16 hours on a regular basis (if using the 16/8 method of fasting) did lose fat but maintained their muscle mass (8).

It is also theorized that intermittent fasting, which can increase growth hormones short-term, may increase your metabolic rate. Further research is needed to validate this theory.

There are some who speculate that intermittent fasting may have anti-aging effects. These were done with rat models and it was found that they lived 36%–83% longer (8). Of course, many of the studies have been for short periods of time, and in some cases there have been no human studies to validate these claims. Of course, more research needs to be done on humans to get a better understanding of how intermittent fasting affects adults.

Who Should Avoid Intermittent Fasting?

Intermittent fasting is not for everyone. Additionally, if you are planning to try this type of lifestyle change or any other lifestyle changes, you should be checking with your doctor to make sure you are healthy and there are no other precautions that need to be taken.

Persons that should avoid this type of lifestyle change include children and teenagers less than the age of 18. In these age groups, teenagers may eat sporadically and may not be able to be disciplined enough to eat specific foods at specific times on a regular basis. Women who are trying to conceive should definitely not try this type of lifestyle change. Since you're eating for two, you need to have the nutrients available on a regular basis and not fast for long periods of time (8).

It goes without saying that persons with a history of eating disorders (anorexia or bulimia) should not even entertain this type of lifestyle change, period. This is because of the distorted eating habits that they have to start with.

Persons who have already been diagnosed with certain diseases such as diabetes should also avoid intermittent fasting. This is due to the fact that some persons with diabetes have a certain amount of carbohydrates and protein they need to consume with each meal. This is very important if they are on insulin (8). Fasting for long periods of time may contribute to higher blood sugar. Please discuss this or any other type of lifestyle change with your doctor; of course persons who have irregular menses should definitely not start this type of lifestyle change. This may increase the irregularity of their menses also.

With the exception of the above-named conditions, intermittent fasting has a very good safety profile. Those who have been screened by their doctors are usually in very good health and they can continue on with intermittent fasting indefinitely. It can be a permanent lifestyle change. Also remember that intermittent fasting may have different effects on different people. If you are experiencing any unusual anxiety, headaches, nausea, or other symptoms after starting intermittent fasting, please contact your doctor (8).

CHAPTER 5

DO I NEED TO EXERCISE?

In addition to finding the right diet that works for you, exercise will help you lose even more weight. I would like to give you first-hand knowledge about why exercise is beneficial. Gone are the days when you're doing this same old exercise all the time and you don't feel like you're making any headway. I have other solutions for you, and you may really enjoy exercise. Besides, we know that there are many beneficial things that exercise can do for us. It does not matter the age, sex, or physical ability. We can all gain something from doing vigorous exercise.

Weight Control

Exercise can prevent excess weight from coming back. The temptation is always to start eating more calories after we've lost the weight. With life's circumstances pulling us in various directions, we can find ourselves gaining weight back. Maintaining an exercise regimen is important to keeping our weight down. You do not have to be in a gym to get these benefits. There are many exercise routines we can get on cable, YouTube, or on the Internet. Also, many of these are free. You can also burn calories by being more active throughout the day. Taking the stairs instead of taking the elevator. Additionally, we can park a further distance away in the parking lot when we get to work. This will enable us to add more walking into our place of business (9).

Improving Health Conditions

There are many diseases that we routinely recommend people to exercise for. This can be depression, anxiety, or other chronic diseases. Among them we would include diabetes mellitus. All too often, people who have diabetes have gained a lot of weight and are not getting better control over their diabetes, which requires them to lose some weight. Losing weight also helps them prevent complications of their disease such as heart disease, stroke, and kidney disease. Heart disease is another health condition that exercise will improve. If you have had a heart attack or you have known heart problems, many cardiologists will ask you to start an exercise program. They know that losing the weight will decrease some of their risk factors. They also know that people feel much better when they're exercising (10).

Diabetes can be one of these health problems. There have been several studies that have shown that a change in diet, exercise, and weight loss can help prevent diabetes. This has been replicated at least three times and the conclusions have been the same. Diet with exercise does a better job of preventing this disorder than just taking medications. Exercise, particularly walking, also helps with balance in the older age groups and it helps prevent patients from having a lot of falls (9).

Improved Mood

Physical activity can stimulate the brain to produce chemicals called endorphins. These chemicals can leave you feeling happier, more relaxed, and less anxious. Persons have also reported that exercise boosts their confidence and improves their self-esteem (9).

Better Energy, Better Sleep

When you start to exercise on a regular basis, your cardiovascular system works more efficiently. You are taking in more oxygen and that appears to increase energy. If you are consistent on a regular basis, you will have more energy than you ever thought you could have.

Many people have problems getting to sleep and staying asleep. Vigorous exercise will solve this problem for a lot of people. You will fall asleep much faster and you will sleep soundly and be refreshed when you get up in the morning (9).

Boosting Your Sex Life

Studies have shown that regular exercise by women can increase their sexual arousal. Men too can benefit from regular exercise. It has been found that men who exercise on a regular basis have less problems with erectile dysfunction than those who do not (9).

Types of Exercise

We have talked about exercise and its benefits. Fortunately, there are many different exercises that we can do to help us with our weight loss and for enjoyment too.

There are national recommendations for the amount of exercise that should be done every week. The CDC recommendation is to do at least 150 minutes a week (12). Many people who have not exercised before can probably not do the 150 minutes but should work their way up to this amount over a period of time. To reach your goals for weight loss, if you are overweight or obese, you may want to try doing a minimum of 250 minutes of moderate-intensity exercise on a weekly basis. If you feel that you want to take your exercise to the next level, try going up to 300 minutes of exercise a week.

Walking Briskly

Walking is the exercise of choice to get started. It is low-impact, and most people can include walking on a daily basis. We're not talking about strolling. In other words, you should not be talking on your cell phone while you're walking. You should have a dedicated time to do continuous walking for a minimum of 30 minutes. You can also do other things to increase the amount of walking you do on a daily basis such as taking the stairs instead of the elevator. You may also try walking around the building several times before work starts (that is, if it is safe). But I must add, you will get the most benefit from continuous walking.

Cycling

This is a very popular exercise that improves your overall fitness and can help you lose weight. You have the option of doing this inside or outside. If you're an outside person, there are usually trails that may be available to you in nearby areas of the city. For those who do not know how to ride a bike, you can always do cycling in a gym class. Either way, you're going to burn calories. Cycling is great for all fitness levels. (This is true whether you are a beginner, have moderate experience, or advanced experience). It is low-impact and non-weight bearing. Studies have shown that people who cycle have over-all better fitness.

Swimming

Swimming is an excellent way to get overall fitness, as it is low impact and easy on the joints. It is also excellent for losing weight. The good thing is you may not have to exercise as much if you do this at least two or three times a week. So, the thing that you need to take into consideration is the fact that you need to learn how to swim (if you do not have the skill already). Also, you need the availability of a pool on a regular basis so that you can continue your exercise. In some areas of the country, pools are not as easily accessible.

Jogging or Running

Jogging and running are great exercises to help you lose weight. These exercises may appear to be similar but there are some differences. Jogging is a much slower-paced exercise, about four to six miles an hour. So, in 30 minutes that will be about two miles. This is assuming you are jogging four miles per hour. Running, on the other hand, is about six to eight miles or more per hour. Many studies show that jogging or running can burn excess belly fat (some would like to characterize it as a muffin top). This is the type of fat that is linked to heart disease and diabetes. Unfortunately, jogging and running can be hard on your joints. You can get around this by using a treadmill or running on grass if possible.

HIIT

A new form of exercise to burn off fat that is very popular in fitness studios and online exercise routines is HIIT. The initials stand for high intensity interval training. These workouts "generally combine short bursts of intense exercise with periods of rest and low-intensity exercise" (11). This type of exercise can result in the body burning calories at a high rate for about 48 to 72 hours later. Since this increases your metabolic rate it helps you burn more calories. This type of exercise can only be done for one to three days a week in order for your body to have time to heal and rest. It is recommended that you start this type of exercise in a class or with a trainer, so you make sure you're doing it at the right intensity and the right amount of time.

Beyond Routine Exercise

This section is for those who have found their passion in running, jogging, swimming, and cycling and want to take their exercising to the next level. I have coached many of my patients to exercise to lose weight and many have wanted to challenge themselves even further. First, I recommend that you talk with your doctor to make sure that you are physically able to participate in strenuous exercise. Many of the races that you can participate in are fundraisers for cancer research, Alzheimer's disease, the American Heart Association, or juvenile diabetes, to mention a few. There are many race types such as 5Ks (or 5000 meters); this about 3.1 miles. If you have gotten up to 45 minutes three to four times a week this would be ideal for you.

These races have gotten very popular and after completing several 5K races, many want to challenge themselves to a 10K type race. This race is about 6.2 miles. Many YMCA's may have training for this; also some stores that sell high-end running shoes may sponsor training. Certain stores that sell high-end sneakers will instruct you on the correct running techniques. In many instances, patients find that these races help them keep weight off. Additionally, many invite friends and family and make it an outing for everyone.

Some of my patients have gone on to do half-marathons and marathons. These types of long-distance races are not for the faint of heart. Many who undertake these races have prior successes with short-term races. Additionally, they have also gotten training on how to pace themselves and how to successfully prepare for these types of races.

What About Our Children?

Our children love to be a part of many things that we participate in. Participation by our children sets up good habits for them as they grow up. Most of the time this can be very fun-filled. Be creative in ways that you introduce exercise to them. You will be creating memories that they will never forget.

I had the opportunity to take care of a wonderful mother and daughter. Marien came to talk to me about weight loss and I gave her a lot of coaching and encouraged her in her efforts. As she started to be successful in her weight loss, I suggested she join one of the exercise groups in the area. In both of these groups, they encouraged their members to join long-distance races. One of these races was the Cooper River Bridge Run. It is about five miles and it is in Charleston, SC. I do recall that participating in the Cooper River Bridge Run was a long-term goal for Marien. She postponed it the year before due to family matters. On one particular occasion in the early fall after her race, Marien came to my office for her routine visit. After the usual greetings, she asked her daughter to tell me what she had done earlier in the summer. Her daughter enthusiastically jumped up and told me that she had accompanied her mother and she ran the five miles at the Cooper River Bridge Run. Marien's daughter was only 13 at the time. This young girl was smiling from ear to ear as she talked about the things that they had encountered on the bridge. This accomplishment was significant for her.

When her daughter was starting school, Marien realized that her daughter needed a lot more support academically. This proved to be very challenging. Eventually Marien settled on a new school, and her young daughter seemed to be more comfortable at this new school. The Cooper River Bridge Run shows that young teenagers need to have all kinds of opportunities to express themselves. Everyone may not be academically inclined but accomplishments like this can improve self-esteem and their confidence. How many young teens that you know could write a story about one of their greatest accomplishments in the year? How many could actually say they had run a five-mile race in the Cooper River Bridge Run? What a profound legacy this mother has left for her child.

CHAPTER 6

STRENGTH TRAINING: ISN'T THIS FOR BODY BUILDERS?

Many people who start on an exercise regimen only do cardio exercise to burn calories. They mistakenly believe that cardio is the best way to lose weight. (It is "one" of the ways to lose weight.) Strength training, on the other hand, helps you burn calories long after you have stopped your workout.

Strength training, also called resistance training, involves using your own body (or with the aid of dumbbells, kettle-bells, or resistance bands, to name a few) to build muscle mass and strength (12).

Many people are not aware of this little-known fact, but weightlifting increases bone density. This recommendation is often given to women starting at about age 50. Many women lose muscle mass at this time and their bone density starts to decline after menopause. Weekly strength or weight training from 20 to 30 minutes two to three times a week helps bone density get to its optimal levels. Additionally, strengthening muscles will make you strong enough to break a fall if this should happen to you. Balance is also a major problem as we get older. Continued strength training ameliorates this condition as people get older (13).

As we consistently do strength training, we enable our muscle mass to increase. As a result of this, your metabolic rate increases. Increased metabolic rate simply means that at rest your body burns more calories. If you are diligent about your weightlifting your metabolic rate will increase and you will burn more calories when you are resting.

At this juncture, it is probably time to give some basic definitions. When reading about strength training you will find references to "reps" and "sets." Reps refers to short repetitions. It is how many times you do a specific exercise (for example, biceps curls). Sets are how many repetitions you do in a row. Of course, you will have periods of rest between the sets.

Example: you may start out with five-pound dumbbells and want to do 8 reps. But you will do two sets. The total number of reps will be 16 when you complete this specific exercise (13).

When beginning your strength training, always do warm-up exercises. Try stretching your hamstrings, calf muscles, and shoulders to start. You may also want to include light cardio for 5 to 10 minutes to warm up your muscles. Start with light weights. I recommend 3 to 5 pounds to start. If these weights feel too light or too easy as you are doing your sets, go up to 5 to 8 pounds. Start with the weights that you feel most comfortable with. Do not push yourself to exhaustion. Many people feel they want to have the fine, defined muscles when they first start out. The person that you see in the gym has been doing that for many years. Also remember to increase your "reps" after about two weeks. If this is your first time using weights, you may want to get a trainer or go to a strengthening class (13).

I must admit I was one of those people that thought that cardio was the only way to go to lose weight. I was introduced to weightlifting in my jazzercise class. They had decided to start a strength training program on the Saturday mornings that I came on a regular basis. I started out with lightweight dumbbells, about three pounds, and gradually increased dumbbells weights as I got stronger. Additionally, I was not aware of all the benefits of strength training when I first started. Shortly thereafter I had to fly to a conference. Much to my surprise, I was actually able to lift up my luggage without any help. I would highly recommend strength training for every woman who is losing weight or wants to stay strong. Additionally, women do tend to lose muscle mass as they get older and that is another reason why strength training is highly recommended. (13).

CHAPTER 7

HOW CAN I DEVELOP GOOD NUTRITION AND EATING HABITS?

On Being Proactive

There are many habits that we may need to improve upon as we go on our lifestyle journey to be the best that we can be. You have probably always heard that breakfast is the most important meal of the day. However, many people skip it due to poor planning or they do not like that feeling of fullness in their stomach early in the morning. It has been estimated that eating breakfast within the first hour of the day can jumpstart your metabolism for the rest of the day. This can happen even without cardio or strength training.

Eating an inadequate breakfast, we are going to be ravenously hungry and we will eat a lot of the wrong foods. Usually, the first thing that people pick up is simple carbohydrates. They are everywhere. The vending machines are full of them. These carbs are meant to get your energy up and you will probably buy a beverage that has a lot of sugar in it also. The end result is that in two hours you will probably crash because all that sugar will be gone, and you will start feeling irritable and grumpy. Be proactive about your breakfast and other meals. I am familiar with this. I have been there!

Lunch presents a different kind of problem. Sometimes meetings are called that you were not aware of. All of a sudden, you panic because you are eating foods that are not part of your lifestyle. Those same machines are there ready for you to purchase what is in there (usually cakes, cookies, candies, chips, and crackers). The other question you may ask yourself is: how long will I be able to work on a pack of crackers and a soda? Your boss may ask you to get the proposal ready today as opposed to next week. How much energy are you going to have? And what is this going to do to your weight loss efforts? Everybody is probably going to order something nearby. But that may not be what your diet is calling for. But you may have no choice if you're going to have to work later in the evening.

Lunch should also be preplanned. Most people usually do it the night before. Usually, it's a sandwich, deli meat and cheese with lettuce and tomato of some sort. This is really good because at least you know what is in the sandwich. You may also want to take a salad along with you because that adds more fiber and actually gives you more green leafy vegetables. Fast food alternatives could also include salads. Many restaurants have beefed up their salad offerings. As usual, please be careful about the calorie content of some of these dressings. I have seen that on occasion the dressing has more calories than the vegetables themselves. And of course, you probably want to do a vinaigrette or a low-calorie dressing.

Dinner is usually at home, and if you're on a diet or changing your lifestyle, most of that should be done or preprepared at home. At least you know what's in the meals that you're preparing. You control how much fat, sugar, and calories you will be getting. I do realize that there are times when it's not possible to eat at home all the time. One easy thing to do is to have the proteins already cooked and packaged in the freezer. This makes it very easy to add vegetables and your favorite carb such as brown rice or sweet potatoes. Additionally, there are subscriptions you can get for prepared meal plans that you can purchase. Just make sure they meet the calorie standards you have for each meal.

Eating Out with a New Lifestyle

Eating out can also present challenges when we're trying to maintain new lifestyle habits and new food choices. You may be wondering, "How can I go with my friends and family and not get this feeling that I'm falling off the wagon?"

Appetizers are ways that restaurants add on to the cost of your meal. The appetizers are absolutely delicious. With your newfound lifestyle changes, you have to decide if you want to add this on. You may figure out which calories would be best for you. I have known people to eat two appetizers and that will be their meal. Also, if one of the appetizers is one of your favorites, just share it with family and friends. If you're watching your calories, you may want to forgo this; just have a salad or a soup.

Breads and rolls find themselves on your table at most restaurants. If your waitress or waiter is on their toes they will wait until the hot bread and rolls come out and you will be able to have melted butter on them. For many people this is very hard to resist. I am one of these people. One way to get around this is to make sure you're not very hungry before coming into the restaurant. For those of you who have built up extreme willpower, it may be easy for you to tell the waitress not to bring any rolls at all. This is a hard choice.

Most restaurants have menus available with the calories for each entree on the menu. Other restaurants have menus that include the carb, fat, and salt content. Still others have what they call a light menu or a light fare menu. This makes it easy to choose something that you know is low in calories. Some of them may be remakes of their regular menu but lower in calories. If the restaurant that you have chosen does not indicate the calories or other nutritional content, order your entree and just ask for a to-go box. You can then eat half of your meal in the restaurant and then you can take the other half with you home. So, you have effectively cut your calories in half for each meal.

You have been sticking to your new lifestyle changes. Since you have been doing such a good job, you have decided to have a cheat meal. Dessert may be high on your list. This can be a very satisfying way of rewarding yourself for all the hard work you have been putting in. It does not make any sense to deprive yourself. But do everything in moderation. Most desserts are very large and too big for most people to eat alone. So, often it's made to be shared with other friends and family. This way you are not overeating, but you are tasting some of the desserts you have not had in quite some time. This is an even better bonus especially if it's your birthday or you're celebrating a happy occasion.

Of course, do not go to all-you-can-eat restaurants. You are guaranteed to overeat, and you will not feel good about yourself. Stay clear of these restaurants. Most restaurants have portion sizes that are more than adequate. Also, you will not be beating yourself up about how much food you ate.

What to Do if You Do Not Have Time

Fortunately, the food industry has heard your concerns. They have prepared breakfast meals already in the freezer section for you. You may have seen boiled eggs in the refrigerator section of your supermarket. You can take these with you and have them for breakfast when you get to work. They also have frozen egg-like mini soufflés that you just microwave according to directions. Some have egg with bacon, ham, or sausage in a little muffin container. Of course, there are many fast-food restaurants that offer breakfast. Just make sure you know the calorie and fat content and how many carbs it has. Many places have a lot of carbohydrates and a lot of fat, which equals a lot of calories. Other suggestions for breakfast may include yogurt or a smoothie that you take with you. Maybe have a boiled egg when you get to work. Protein bars are also a good alternative. This is so that you can get the energy you need and reduce carbohydrates you would get from the vending machine products. This is definitely a better alternative. If you are going to have boxed cereals, make sure it is high in fiber (4 grams or more); this will keep you full and satisfied. You may have this with regular milk or almond, soy, or oat milk (there are so many types of milks, I cannot keep up with them). In summary, there are many fast-food restaurants that offer breakfast. Just be sure you know the nutritional content. There is usually a lot of fat and carbohydrates in these meals. Eating half of a sandwich can also be an alternative for breakfast and take some yogurt and/or a smoothie with you. Always keep protein bars on hand as a snack just for those times that you get hungry.

For lunch, the sandwich is a good staple. Make sure you use bread that has whole wheat flour as the first ingredient. Always make sure this bread has a minimum of 2 grams of fiber per slice. You can add a salad or bring additional veggies with you. Bagged salads are easy to take along; just bring your own low-calorie dressing.

Dinner is usually the heaviest meal of the day. Make sure you have good nutrition and fiber with this meal. Usually, 2–3 oz. of protein for women and 4–5 oz. of protein for men. Make sure you eat a lot of veggies (about a cup), and brown rice, quinoa, sweet potatoes, or another carb. It is good to have salad with this meal to get more veggies. You may want to add chickpeas to get additional fiber. As was stated before, it is convenient to have prepared protein (chicken, turkey, or beef) cooked and frozen in the freezer. This makes it easy to put a meal together in the evening. If this is one of those days you do not want to cook, a good number of restaurants can prepare one of your favorite entrees for pickup. You can also use Uber or DoorDash. Just remember to do your homework about the nutritional content of the meal so you are not going over your calorie count for the day.

Skipping Meals

If skipping meals is a habit, you are going to need to focus on building in ways to eat regularly. This will increase your success with your weight loss journey. You are going to need to fuel your weight loss. Every few hours you should be eating a meal or a snack. Your body needs to know that it's getting its needed nutrients from the food that you are eating. If your body does not get these needed nutrients, it will stall your weight loss. Many people feel that eating less will help them lose weight. Unfortunately, skipping meals will decrease your metabolic rate (how fast your body burns up calories). I have seen many people starting out very strong on their diet, but due to skipping meals, they had not lost any weight at all. So, it is important that you fuel your weight loss at regular intervals during the day. This will also keep your metabolic rate working efficiently to burn up excess fat you have stored up. As you can see, skipping meals can be counter-productive.

When we skip meals our blood sugar drops; we feel fatigued and irritable. Sometimes we feel angry and moody. This prevents us from being efficient at our tasks and making decisions. As we stated earlier, skipping meals decreases our metabolic rate, thus making it harder for us to lose weight. When you skip a meal, your body goes into survival mode (14). This causes the cells in your body to crave food, which causes you to become ravenously hungry. Guess what, you usually crave carbs and other foods which are not the best foods for you.

There are ways to stave off hunger. Sometimes you have to go to an unscheduled meeting, or you have to pick up the kids unexpectedly. Try keeping high-protein snacks with you or at your office. These high-protein snacks can include yogurt, cheese and crackers, or peanut butter and crackers. You may also want protein bars that have a lot of fiber. Also put an alarm on your cell phone for your next meal so that you can have that time set aside for yourself to eat. As we discussed earlier, preplanning for these times is the best way to prevent going hungry (14).

I have had some personal experience with some of these issues. I have skipped meals and felt like I had to eat everything in sight! Once I started preplanning my meals and snacks, I felt in better control and I was not overeating. I no longer had to figure out what snacks I needed to get from the vending machines. Even with good planning there were occasions that I did go to the local vending machines, but this was the exception rather than the rule. Also, my grumpiness factor went down. I did not have those late-morning hunger spikes. I usually had a protein bar or some other snack at my desk. Hopefully, this may give you some insight into some issues you may be facing.

CHAPTER 8

WHY IS FIBER GOOD FOR MY HEALTH AND LIFESTYLE?

Sonja had been having increasing stomach pain. This had been going on for two weeks. Initially she thought it was gas. She bought at least two containers of Gas-X. This medicine did not help at all. She then went online to see if she could find out the cause of her stomach pain. She found some information that hinted that she may have appendicitis. This was very alarming to her. She started thinking about what would happen if her appendix ruptured. This scared her the most. Her imagination started to run away with her. She started thinking about all the different types of scenarios that could occur. She became so anxious and afraid that she drove herself to the hospital. While there, she was given an IV and they drew her blood for lab work. The doctor who saw her ordered a CT scan of the abdomen. While there, she was busy telling friends on the phone that she may have appendicitis. Finally, at 9:00 PM (she had gotten there about 4:00 in the afternoon) all the tests were back. Fortunately, while the lab work was normal and her CT scan of the abdomen did not show that she had appendicitis, it showed extensive stool in her colon. Essentially, she was constipated. Stool was all through her colon!

She did not believe the doctor when she was told this. How could constipation cause so much pain? She even asked the doctor if he was sure. She was told that this CT scan was a preliminary report and that they would get back to her when the report was finalized. But he said to her that this pattern is very consistent with constipation and he doubted if it is something else. Sonja walked out of the emergency room in disbelief. She could not believe that all this pain was caused by her not having consistent bowel movements.

Let's look at what fiber can do to help us maintain our healthy lifestyles and healthy daily habits.

Dietary fiber has a lot of advantages. One of them is preventing constipation. It can also aid in helping maintain a healthy weight. Fiber is also known to lower your risk of diabetes and some cancers. Dietary fiber is an essential part of a healthy diet and fiber is found in fruits and vegetables, whole grains, and legumes. It also keeps the gut healthy and it reduces the risk of chronic diseases.

Fiber is found in two forms.

Soluble fiber: this type of fiber dissolves in water to form a gel-like substance. It can lower cholesterol and help regulate blood sugar. It is found in oats, peas, beans, apples, and citrus fruits.

Insoluble fiber: this type of fiber helps the passage of food through the digestive tract and increases the bulk in your stools, which is very beneficial to those who have constipation. It's found in whole wheat, flour, ground flax seeds, chia seeds, wheat bran, nuts, and cauliflower, to mention a few options.

Fiber can also help you maintain better health. Fiber is important to keeping the gut healthy. Eating the correct amount of fiber can prevent or relieve constipation, as stated before. Fiber can help the waste in your body move smoothly and quickly through your colon. It also encourages healthy gut microbacteria.

High-fiber diets can lower your risk of developing hemorrhoids and also small pouches from developing along your colon. The small pouches that develop are called diverticular disease. Many people in their 40s and 50s start to get this very painful disease. Foods rich in fiber may also lower your risk of colon cancer (15).

High-fiber foods can aid in maintaining a healthy weight. These foods tend to be more filling than low-fiber foods. This will enable you to eat less and feel satisfied longer (you will not get hungry as quickly). Additionally, high-fiber foods tend to take longer to eat and tend to be "energy dense." This means they have fewer calories for the same volume of food (15).

Research also suggests that increasing dietary fiber may be associated with a reduced risk of dying from cardiovascular disease and from some cancer (16).

Recommendations for Fiber on a Daily Basis

For men and women under the ages of 50:

1. Men should be getting at least 38 grams of fiber per day
2. Women should be getting at least 25 grams of fiber per day

For men and women over age 51:

1. Men should be getting 30 grams of fiber per day
2. Women should be getting 21 grams of fiber per day (15).

During pregnancy or breastfeeding,

1. Women should aim to get 20 grams of fiber a day (16).

Additional Suggestions for Increasing Fiber in Your Diet

At breakfast, choose a high-fiber cereal that has five grams or more per serving. Try to find cereals that list whole grains like oats, wheat, and bran, to name a few. You can also try combining cereals to increase the amount of fiber you get per serving.

Smoothies are another excellent way to get extra fiber. By adding ground flax seeds, chia seeds, or unprocessed bran, you will increase the amount of fiber per day.

Try switching to whole grains. Try to consume half of all your grains as whole grains. Look for breads that have whole wheat, whole wheat flour, or another whole grain as the first ingredient.

Incorporate legumes in your diet, such as black beans, red beans, pigeon peas, and lentils, which are good sources of fiber. Also try to incorporate different types of legumes in your salads. These can include chickpeas or kidney beans.

It is recommended that you increase your fiber amount slowly so that you do not suffer from gas and bloating. Remember, if you're increasing the amount of fiber you eat, please increase your water also. This may mean you'll have to drink more than the recommended eight glasses of water per day. I would aim to get 10–12 glasses of water a day.

You can find fiber in most of your fruits and vegetables. It is good to have at least five servings of fruits and veggies each day. The following is a short list of high-fiber foods. This list can give you some ideas as to how much fiber you will get in your daily diet (16).

Food	Serving size	Calories	Dietary fiber in g
High-fiber bran (ready-to-eat cereal)	1/2–3/4 of a cup	60–81	9.1–14.3
Chickpeas, canned	1/2 a cup	176	8.1
Lentils, cooked	1/2 a cup	115	7.8
Pinto beans, cooked	1/2 a cup	122	7.7
Black beans, cooked	1/2 a cup	114	7.5
Lima beans, cooked	1/2 a cup	108	6.6
White beans, canned	1/2 tha cup	149	6.3
Kidney beans	1/2 a cup	112	5.7
Wheat bran flakes (ready-to-eat cereal)	3/4 of a cup	90–98	4.9–5.5
Raw pear	1 medium fruit	101	5.5
Baked beans, canned, plain	1/2 a cup	119	5.2
Avocado	1/2 a cup	120	5.0
Mixed vegetables, cooked from frozen	1/2 a cup	59	4.0

Food	Serving size	Calories	Dietary fiber in g
Raspberries	1/2 a cup	32	4.0
Blackberries	1/2 a cup	31	3.8
Collards, cooked	1/2 a cup	32	3.8
Sweet potato, baked in skin	1 medium vegetable	103	3.8

CHAPTER 9

WHAT IS THE ART OF RECHARGING

Have you ever planned a much-needed vacation? Maybe you went to one of your favorite vacation spots in the Caribbean. While you were there, you were able to relax and experience all the activities that were available to you. You even signed up for a massage on the beach. There were usually evening activities that you participated in that were a lot of fun. Since this was an all-inclusive resort you were able to go to various restaurants of your choice. Of course, you went to the beach every day. Many times, you sat and watched the sunset. As you were there you felt the stress and the cares of your regular workdays drift away. When you got back, your family and your coworkers commented on how refreshed and relaxed you look from going on this vacation.

Suppose you could have mini recharges and have your mind and body feel recharged on a regular basis. These times that we take out for ourselves help us to cope with life's challenges and stressors.

Rejuvenation refers to refreshing your mind, body, and spirit after or during a busy day. It is an essential part of any exercise program. This is as stated by Greg Hottinger and Michael Scholtz in their book *Coach Yourself Thin* (17). They feel that this is what everyone needs to stay motivated and excited about what they're doing in their weight loss efforts. Additionally, times of rejuvenation will improve your exercise performance and reduce chances of injury.

In attending to these processes, we have to be aware of our emotions and what we're experiencing at the moment they are happening. Knowing there will be challenges in your weight loss program but having the attitude that "I'm going to stick with it until I reach my successful goals" shows an attitude of persistence. You may be going through various emotions even though you're thinking about sticking with it. Also, it is important to listen to your body and know what your strengths and limitations are. This can happen with any endeavor.

In the process of recharging, you will feel comfortable taking a pause and get to some perspective about yourself. This will enable you to review what you have accomplished and plan what you want to accomplish later on with your weight loss goals. The recharging process can occur with different techniques. These are techniques that you can do on a regular basis to recharge yourself. Some may meet your needs and others may not be as important to you.

If you have a job that requires you to sit in front of a computer that is not adjusted to your height, you can get a lot of shoulder and neck pain from strain and stress. You will probably also need to have an ergonomic evaluation to prevent this from happening again. Entailed in that evaluation will be the right types of tools to make you more comfortable at your worksite. You will still need to stretch out those muscles and do self-care to keep those muscles in shape. Headaches may also be a prominent complaint. Exercises that can help these muscles can help you maintain a good range of motion. Exercises like yoga, massage, and Pilates will enable you to accomplish this (17).

Sometimes we need to focus on breathing and engaging in mind-quieting techniques. These techniques have been proven to reduce stress. They also make us aware of how we are feeling and that we have been present in the moment. This enables you to be more contemplative and think clearly about goals and objectives. Doing mindfulness exercises can help with these relaxation techniques. These include autogenic exercises and visual imagery, to name a few. They enable you to move to a state of relaxation and calmness. These exercises, when done regularly, can refresh you and enable you to meet the stresses of life.

There are other forms of relaxation that you can include in your techniques for recharging. Having a nice warm bath at home or getting to a jacuzzi can relax tired muscles and help you recover from stressors that you have been confronted with. I have found that getting a monthly massage can also bring deep relaxation. They are usually done in quiet rooms with relaxing music. After one hour with these massages you can feel like a new person ready to cope with all the challenges that may happen. Although this cannot be done daily, this is just part of your list of techniques to use for relaxation.

Additionally, regular restful sleep has been recommended for everyone. The ability to unwind and have your body reset for the next day is undoubtedly the best way to recharge. The recommendation is to get seven to eight hours of sleep a night. All too often, many people report that they are not able to get this amount of sleep. Sometimes this is because they're not unwinding an hour before they go to bed. It is recommended that you turn off all the screen devices and listen to some soft music. This may indeed help you to relax so that you can fully fall asleep. If you enjoy reading, it is recommended that you use a paper book rather than a Kindle or another screen device. Evidently, the light in these devices has an ability to trigger a wakefulness, which is exactly the opposite of what you want to do. Other things to consider are the temperature in the room and the absence of extra light in the bedroom. These suggestions often work for most people. If you are having difficulty with your sleep, it is probably advisable for you to contact your doctor for further evaluation.

Recharging can make you more settled and energized on a daily basis. Coping and decision-making will come from your ability to think clearly about each individual situation. You will also be more satisfied with what you're accomplishing with your weight loss goals.

PART 2

What Are We Really Eating?

CHAPTER 10

WHAT ARE NATURAL SWEETENERS?

It is known that people in the United States consume much too much sugar on a daily basis. Most of it's from processed food and sugar-sweetened beverages. It is also known that diets high in sugar are linked with obesity, prediabetes, heart disease, and tooth decay. The best way to lower your risk for these disorders is to gradually reduce the amount of sugar you consume on a daily basis. This may take a while but it's worth it. Today we have a lot of artificial sweeteners and some of them have been linked to obesity and diabetes. So, if you would like something sweet you may want to try natural sweeteners.

Stevia

Stevia comes from a plant whose leaves have glycoside compounds. They are three hundred times sweeter than sugar. When using this compound, you do not need much to sweeten your coffee or tea. The sweetener has no effect on blood sugar or insulin. This is important if you're diabetic. You can find this in most stores as Truvia or stevia in the raw (these are just a few of the products available). From personal experience I can say that I have tried quite a few of these commercial types and sometimes they can have an after-taste. I tend to stick to the ones that only have pure stevia. Sometimes stevia is combined with erythritol. You will find this combination quite often. Another combination of stevia is also with dextrose. This flavor combination seems to have an after-taste, so it depends on what you prefer (44).

Monk Fruit

This is another natural sweetener. It is extracted from a melon that comes from Southeast Asia. This, like Stevia, has no impact on your blood sugar. You can find this commercially as monk fruit in the raw. I have tried the sweetener and found it to have a very good flavor, and it does a good job of sweetening your beverages (18).

Agave Syrup

This syrup comes from the agave cactus. The agave nectar is extracted from the cactus, which contains compounds called fructans. These fructans are advantageous in lowering blood sugar.

Unfortunately, when commercial manufacturers process these fructans, they are converted to fructose. So in fact, what you're purchasing is a product that is something similar to high- fructose corn syrup. It is considered a natural sweetener but it is one that should be avoided. I have tried agave also, but I find it to be messy and similar to honey (18).

Sugar Alcohols

These include sorbitol, erythritol, and xylitol. You will find these sugars in yogurt, sugar-free gum, sugar-free candy, etc. They are lower in calories and sugar and do not affect the blood sugar. The sugar-free gum has helped many people decrease the number of cavities that they have. Sugar alcohols are not the sweetest, so you may need to increase the amount to get the correct sweetness level you want. Things to watch out for include bloating, abdominal discomfort, gas, and diarrhea. You may experience all of these symptoms or just one. Xylitol is the sweetest of the group but just be aware that it is toxic to dogs. These are considered a safe choice, but you must limit the amount that you use. This is to avoid the GI side effects that we discussed earlier (18).

High-Fructose Corn Syrup

This sweetener is in almost everything. It does make our food sweeter; it's in most foods and beverages that are sweet. This is because it is very inexpensive to manufacture. This is the number one reason why the consumption has steadily increased year after year. This sugar also has a longer half-life. And this helps stores and people who have storage space at home to keep their goods for longer periods of time. There are several disadvantages, however, to using high- fructose corn syrup. Many people are not aware that they are taking in excess amounts of sugar from soft drinks and processed foods. Remember that any sugar that is not used by the body gets stored as fat in your body. Thus, it will start to increase your weight and it may increase the bad cholesterol, which is the LDL cholesterol. This is a marker for the beginnings of heart disease. This excess stored fat can also get stored in your liver, causing fatty liver disease. Although high- fructose corn syrup is sweeter, hunger is less satisfied by using this sugar. This means that you are only satisfied for shorter periods of time and you will be eating more frequently than you need to. Additionally, farmers are very highly motivated to get these crops to market as soon as possible. To do this they use additional pesticides too, to make sure their crops are insect- and pest-free. This may mean that you're getting additional pesticide residue in your high-fructose corn syrup. Of course, these pesticide residues do not have to be put on any labeling that you may receive for these goods (18).

We have given you just a brief overview of some of the natural sugars you may want to consider in your quest for having a healthier diet and lifestyle. Remember, what you don't know *can* hurt you, and automatically assuming that whatever is on the label is healthy may be a false assumption. Always check the labels to make sure that you're getting healthy, wholesome, and nutritious foods. Likewise, make sure that you're taking in natural products and you know how they were manufactured, thereby boosting your health in many ways.

CHAPTER 11

WHY SHOULD I AVOID CERTAIN PRESERVATIVES?

There are many foods in our supermarkets that contain preservatives. Some of them we cannot even fully pronounce. Many people wrongfully assume that the FDA is regulating them. The FDA has deemed them as being safe and therefore can be put in certain foods. These preservatives are usually placed in highly processed foods. Also, they may have harmful effects on our bodies. Because these are in highly processed foods most of the time, the nutritional value is questionable. I feel that since we are making some healthy changes to our diets, at this point it is good to know what preservatives are found in certain foods.

Benzoate is listed as a dietary supplement and it is one of the most common food preservatives. It can cause allergies and it's found in carbonated drinks, fruit juices, flour, and beer.

Mono- and diglycerides are a permitted additive in many foods. They are emulsifiers, which prevent water and oil from separating. They do contain small amounts of trans fat. Eating large amounts of these trans fats can be harmful. They have been linked to heart attacks and strokes. Additionally, many foods with other emulsifiers also contain saturated fats. These emulsifiers may not be completely labeled. So, you may want to avoid them.

Propyl gallate is found in meat products, microwave popcorn, soup mixes, mayonnaise, and frozen meals. It works to stop oxygen molecules from mixing with oil in food. This prevents the food from becoming rancid. It may cause stomach and skin irritations, and in the past it has been known to cause kidney and liver problems. It is suggested that you read the labels and avoid this preservative.

Sodium nitrite and sodium nitrate are found in preserved meats and they give them a nice color. These are usually found in hot dogs, bacon, and ham. These chemicals are used to preserve shelf life. Once these meats get cooked, the nitrates convert to nitrosamines, which are associated with an increased risk of certain cancers. Fortunately, there are newer preserved meats on the market that do not contain these preservatives. They may be marked in your meat section as uncured meats. They do have some salt but they do not have these extra chemicals. When you're storing them in the refrigerator, you need to keep in mind how soon you're going to use them (remember, these products have a shorter shelf life). You may need to store them in the freezer if you are not going to use your supply immediately.

BHA and BHT (butylated hydroxyanisole and butylated hydroxytoluene) extend shelf life. They also keep foods from becoming rancid. Both of these preservatives have been deemed potentially carcinogenic to humans. They are found in a number of products including cereal, sausages, hot dogs, and beer, to name a few (19).

Potassium bromate is a food preservative used to increase the volume in breads and rolls. It has been banned in several countries because it has been shown to cause cancer in animal models. It is found most commonly in breads and flours. It is important to read the labels when you purchase foods containing this preservative.

Artificial sweeteners have been on the market for many years now. These are products that were specifically developed for diabetic patients who cannot use regular sugar. Since they do not raise blood sugar, many people thought they were a panacea for eating something sweet. These sweeteners also do not add calories. Many of these artificial sweeteners are believed to be carcinogenic. Some people actually have headaches and digestive problems as a result of taking these sweeteners. But they can also trick your brain into forgetting that sweetness might mean extra calories. Many people actually eat more over time. Thus, they are gaining weight and do not realize it. These artificial sweeteners have also been known to release insulin even though you are eating artificial sweeteners. This may ultimately change the insulin response in your body. These ingredients are found in many products, from sugar-free sodas, gum, yogurt, and desserts to toothpaste. This is not an exhaustive list. If you are looking for something that is a sweetener, try some of the natural sweeteners that we have discussed.

Monosodium glutamate (MSG) is a flavor enhancer that contains an amino acid. Regular consumption of monosodium glutamate has been shown to stimulate your appetite and contribute to weight gain and obesity. Some people have been known to get headaches actually in Chinese restaurants while they're eating this preservative. There are many Chinese restaurants that have decreased or eliminated MSG. It is found in canned meats, frozen goods, salad dressings, chips, and canned soups.

RGH and rBST stand for recombinant bovine growth hormone and recombinant bovine somatotropin hormone. These growth hormones are designed to boost milk production in dairy cows. Milk from cows that are given these growth hormones have high levels of insulin, like growth factor (IGF-D). Breast cancer, colon cancer, and prostate cancer have been associated with this hormone. It is also found that it can create certain types of infections in these large dairy farms, thus necessitating the farmers having to treat the dairy cows with large amounts of antibiotics. There is no labeling required for these hormones. Of note, this hormone has been banned in several countries, including Canada. To find a healthy alternative look for products that say no RGB H or no RBST.

Artificial food colorings are used to make food look bright and colorful. These food colorings have been banned in Europe for many years. This is because they have been found to be linked to various cancers, chromosomal damage, and behavioral problems such as ADD and hyperactivity in children. These are found in quite a few products, including pie mixes, ice cream, candy, mac and cheese, and American cheese. They are also found in puddings and jams. This is not an exhaustive list.

Trans fats and hydrogenated vegetable oils are many products that we purchase on a regular basis. Trans fats are created when regular fats like corn soy or palm oil are commercially changed by adding hydrogen bonds. This makes the liquid oils a solid compound. This process helps them have a longer shelf life. These fats have contributed to raising LDL levels, which is the bad cholesterol, and it lowers the good cholesterol, the HDL levels. These compounds have been actively linked to heart disease, obesity, strokes, and other metabolic disorders. They are found in deep-fried foods, margarines, chips, crackers, and fast foods (20).

EPILOGUE

I hope this book has given you many ideas on how to start your new weight loss journey— the journey that does not carry the baggage that you carried before when you were trying to lose weight. This is a new time, a new age, and new circumstances. And this book has many different ways for you to approach your weight loss. There are many options available to you that do include a regular physician or health coach. Health coaches may be a better opportunity for you because they are singularly-minded in helping you get to your weight loss goal. Additionally, we are more forthright in explaining how mindset plays a major role in many pursuits that are successful. As we stated, a positive mindset will take you much further and almost guarantee success. It does require that you be persistent and give yourself some time to reach the goal that you intended. Take along with you your family and your friends who are your support system. Be encouraged by these cheerleaders who want to see you succeed. Keep in mind that we want you to make a lifestyle change, not just lose weight. As you know, all too often people feel that once they have lost the weight, they return to the same eating habits that created the excess weight. This will not give you the long-term results that you desire.

I wish you success with your new weight loss journey, and always keep in mind that health coaches may be the answer at this point in your life.

ACKNOWLEDGMENTS

This is for all of my patients who accepted my weight loss challenge. This is for all who have started exercising and have completed your first 5K or 10K. This is for all of my patients who stuck with their program even though it was difficult. This is for all of my patients who thought that you wanted to do more and went on to start running on a regular basis. This is for all of my patients who decided that a different lifestyle was the best thing that you ever did. I would like to thank you for giving me the privilege of working with you.

REFERENCES

Chapter 1

(1) "Weight-Loss Readiness," Mayo Clinic, March 22, 2019, https://www.mayoclinic.org/healthy-lifestyle/weight-loss/in-depth/weight-loss/art-20044199.

Chapter 2

(2) "Mind Matters: How to Effortlessly Have More Positive Thoughts," tLEX Institute, accessed March 18, 2021. https://tlexinstitute.com/how-to-effortlessly-have-more-positive-thoughts/.

(3) K. Aleisha Fetters, MS, CSCS, "10 Ways to Shift Your Mindset for Better Weight Loss," U.S. News, accessed March 18, 2021, https://health.usnews.com/wellness/articles/2016-09-19/10-ways-to-shift-your-mindset-for-better-weight-loss.

Chapter 3

(4) Hallie Gould, "3 Popular Diets That Actually Work (and 3 That Don't)," Byrdie, March 8, 2021, https://www.byrdie.com/popular-diets.

(5) "What Is Keto Diet?" U.S. News, January 2, 2019, https://health.usnews.com/best-diet/keto-diet.

(6) Karen Asp, "WW (Formerly Called Weight Watchers),"
WebMD, accessed March 19, 2019, https://www.webmd.com/
diet/a-z/weight-watchers-diet.

(7) Tosca Reno, *The Eat-Clean Diet*, 2007.

Chapter 4

(8) "Intermittent Fasting: What Is It, and How Does It Work?,"
Johns Hopkins Medicine, accessed March 19, 2021, https://
www.hopkinsmedicine.org/health/wellness-and-prevention/
intermittent-fasting-what-is-it-and-how-does-it-work; Kris
Gunnars, BSc, "Intermittent Fasting 101 — The Ultimate
Beginner's Guide," healthline, April 20, 2020, https://www.
healthline.com/nutrition/intermittent-fasting-guide.

Chapter 5

(9) Mayo Clinic Staff, "Exercise: 7 Benefits of Regular Physical Activity," Mayo Clinic, accessed March 19, 2021, https://
www.mayoclinic.org/healthy-lifestyle/fitness/in-depth/
exercise/art-20048389.

(10) "Exercise & Fitness," Harvard Health Publishing,
accessed March 19, 2021, https://www.health.harvard.edu/
topics/exercise-and-fitness.

(11) Julia Belluz, "How to Get the Most Out of Your Exercise
Time, According to Science," accessed March 19, 2021, https://
www.vox.com/science-and-health/2019/1/10/18148463/
high-intensity-interval-training-hiit-orangetheory.

(12) "How Much Physical Activity Do Adults Need?," Centers for Disease Control and Prevention, accessed 03/19/2021, https://www.cdc.gov/physicalactivity/basics/adults/index.htm.

Chapter 6

(13) Jasmine Gomez, "Strength Training 101: How to Get Started," Women's Health, January 23, 2020, https://www.womenshealthmag.com/fitness/a30522035/what-is-strength-training/.

Chapter 7

(14) "What Happens to the Body When You Skip Meals?," accessed March 19, 2021, https://www.piedmont.org/living-better/what-happens-to-the-body-when-you-skip-meals.

Chapter 8

(15) Mayo Clinic Staff, "Dietary Fiber: Essential for a Healthy Diet," Mayo Clinic, January 6, 2021, https://www.mayoclinic.org/healthy-lifestyle/nutrition-and-healthy-eating/in-depth/fiber/art-20043983.

(16) Tim Newman, "Why Do We Need Dietary Fiber?," Medical News Today, April 27, 2020, https://www.medicalnewstoday.com/articles/146935.

Chapter 9

(17) Greg Hottinger, MPH, RD, and Michael Scholtz, MA, *Coach Yourself Thin: Five Steps to Retrain Your Mind, Reclaim Your Power, and Lose the Weight for Good*, 2011.

Chapter 10

(18) Cathe Friedrich, "The Pros and Cons of Various Natural Sweeteners," cathe, accessed March 19, 2021, https://cathe.com/the-pros-and-cons-of-various-natural-sweeteners/.

Chapter 11

(19) "7 Food Preservatives You Should Avoid," Chicago Internal Cleansing, accessed March 19, 2021, https://chicagointernalcleansing.com/7-food-preservatives-you-should-avoid/.

(20) Anjali Shah, "The Top Five Worst Preservatives in Processed Food," The Picky Eater, June 24, 2020, https://pickyeaterblog.com/worst-food-preservatives/.

ABOUT THE AUTHOR

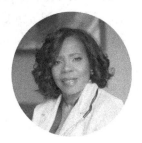

Dr. Hope Watts is a board-certified family physician, health coach, speaker, and lifestyle expert. She is passionate about bringing insight to weight loss struggles. In her many years of practice, she has helped women achieve their lifestyle goals through positive proper diet and exercise and positive mindset.

Dr. Watts earned her undergraduate degree from Temple University and her medical degree from the Medical College of Pennsylvania. Bothe schools are in Philadelphia Pennsylvania. She completed her residency at Saint Francis Hospital in Wilmington, Delaware. Dr. Watts is a Fellow of the American Academy of Family Physicians and the Medical Director of Espera W LLC. She was nominated for the Physician of the Year Award in 2007 by Novant Health Presbyterian Hospital. She has also had additional certification for Diabetes which was given by the National Committee for Quality Assurance. This certification indicates adherence to national guidelines for diabetic care. She was also given an award by Novartis for one of their products that helped her hypertensive patients.

Dr. Watts currently resides in North Carolina, and enjoys bike riding, traveling, exercising, and dancing.

To connect, follow her on social media or email her at info@drhopewatts.com

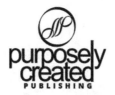

CREATING DISTINCTIVE BOOKS
WITH INTENTIONAL RESULTS

We're a collaborative group of creative masterminds with a mission to produce high-quality books to position you for monumental success in the marketplace.

Our professional team of writers, editors, designers, and marketing strategists work closely together to ensure that every detail of your book is a clear representation of the message in your writing.

Want to know more?
Write to us at info@publishyourgift.com
or call (888) 949-6228

Discover great books, exclusive offers, and more at
www.PublishYourGift.com

Connect with us on social media

@publishyourgift

CPSIA information can be obtained
at www.ICGtesting.com
Printed in the USA
BVHW040714280721
613015BV00019B/687

9 781644 843840